The
Art Of
CBD
Hemp Oil

The Beginner's Guide to Using CBD Hemp Oil to Reduce Pain and Cure Illnesses (Arthritis, Acne, Diabetes, Fibromyalgia)

Table of Contents

Get Your Free Gift!

Are you interested in learning more about Alternative Medicine and how to start using herbal remedies, acupressure or do aromatherapy to achieve long and healthy lifestyle?
You are on the right place!

I giveaway this bundle of 3 totally free books that will reveal everything you need to know to achieve a healthy lifestyle and live a long and happy life! The bundle won't be up forever, so get it before it's taken down. It's my simple way of saying thank you for reading my book.
https://www.subscribepage.com/freebooksonalternativemedicine

Download one of the BEST Bundles **ABSOLUTELY FREE** that will help you learn more about Alternative Medicine.

Introduction

If you are searching for a comprehensive CBD oil guide then you have landed in the right place. If you want a vibrant skin, fight depression, cure chronic pain, lower inflammation or stop the growth of cancer cells, then the CBD oil is your answer. The book covers all that you need to know about CBD oil in order to master your own medical treatment. The health benefits of CBD oil are well established and so many people are now turning to it to cope with pain and diseases. What separates this book from the rest is the fact that you will find all the information on how to properly use the CBD oil for a variety of health issues. This Ultimate Beginner's Guide on CBD Oil will help you understand the topic better, so you know how to safely use CBD for your own health.

.Chapter 1 What is CBD Hemp Oil?

CBD Hemp Oil

CBD Hemp oil or Cannabidiol Hemp Oil is a cannabinoid. Cannabidiol (CBD) is a chemical compound that comes from the hemp plant. It is one of over 85 unique compounds found in hemp. Cannabidiol Hemp Oil is a biologically active cannabis compound that has been proven to have numerous health benefits. The cannabis plant is composed of a complex chemical mixture that includes steroids, flavonoids, terpenoids, phytocannabinoids, and enzymes. Tetrahydrocannabinol (THC) and cannabidiol (CBD) are the two most abundant cannabinoids found naturally in hemp and studied extensively. Most of us already know about tetrahydrocannabinol (THC), the 'high' ingredient in marijuana; but the focus is now shifting to CBD.

THC is the psychoactive component, which causes you to get 'high'. On the other hand, CBD is non-psychoactive, meaning it does not make people 'high or stoned' (https://www.ncbi.nlm.nih.gov/pmc/articles/PMC3797438/). So you can use CBD oil and perform daily tasks such as working, taking care of children and driving without risking yourself or others. CBD oil is an appealing option for people looking for relief from various conditions such as spasms, seizures, psychosis, anxiety, pain, and inflammation. CBD was first isolated in the 1930s and in the 1940s. However, it was Professor Raphael Mechoulam and his team who decoded its structure and configuration in the 1960s.

Cannabidiols originate in marijuana and hemp variations of cannabis. The CBD produced from hemp is legal in the U.S. because it only contains a slight amount of THC. However, CBD found in marijuana is federally illegal in the United States except in specific states. You can purchase CBD hemp oil products in the form of daily capsules, drops, chewing gum and high concentration extracts. Also, some skin creams and shampoos contain this product.

CBD oils healthy ingredients include

- o   Omega 3 fatty acids

- o   Omega 6 fatty acids

- o   Hemp proteins

- o   Vitamin B

- o   Vitamin E

- o   Carotene

CBD oil at a glance

- o   Chemical compound extracted from the Cannabis Sativa L. Plant o   Belongs to a group of molecules known as cannabinoids

o   Nutrient-rich hemp contains essential fatty acids and excellent nutritional value

o   Non- Psychotoxic

o   Supports balance in the endocannabinoid system

o   Legal dietary supplement

Let's go into a deeper discussion on how CBD oil helps your body. From the following discussion, you will know why using CBD oil is so beneficial for the human body.

Understanding the master control system, also known as the Endocannabinoid system.

o   A collection of endogenous cannabinoid receptors positioned all over the central, and tangential nervous systems, and the mammalian brain.

o   Directly involved in regulating mood, sensation, intraocular pressure, appetite, metabolic health, thermoregulation, pain/inflammation, muscle control, motivation/reward, and memory.

o   Involved in synaptic plasticity and learning

- o Endocannabinoids are messengers that communicate through cannabinoid receptors

    - Main Receptors: CB1 and CB2

    - Anandamide and 2AG

    - Also, non-CB receptors

Endocannabinoid System Control

- o Endocannabinoid system tone requires CB1 and CB2 balance

- o Optimal CB1 activity decreases inflammation, reduces pain, decreases anxiety, help to manage stress and controls cognitive function and memory.

- o Prolong stress; eating a poor diet can overstimulate CB1 activity.

- o Overstimulation of CB1 has many negative side effects and could cause inflammation, sleep disruption, anxiety, insulin resistance, etc. in the body.

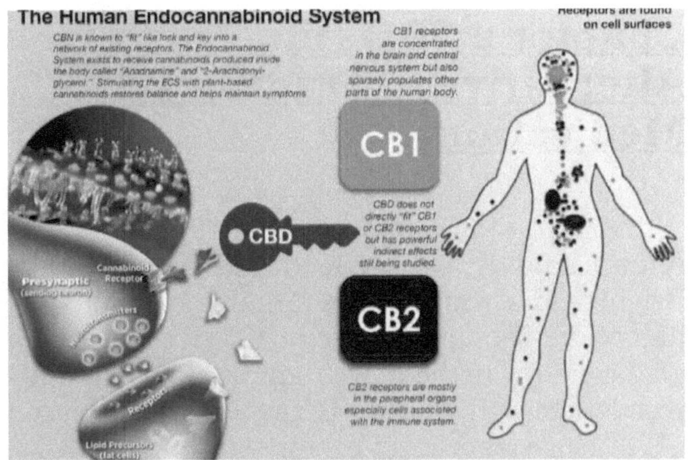

What is CBD oil's role in balancing CB1 and CB2?

CBD can balance the constant overstimulation of the CB1 receptor in several ways.

1. CBD acts as an antagonist to the CB1 receptor

2. It can gently stimulate CB2

3. CBD can stimulate receptors outside of the endocannabinoid system. This helps to modulate inflammation, pain and decrease anxiety.

Essentially, using CBD oil helps balance the system that keeps you balanced. Traditional medications only treat your diseases. On the other hand, CBD oil keeps your system balanced so you stay disease free and this is one of the major differences between traditional medicine and CBD oil.

Chapter 2 CBD Oil: A Better Alternative to Traditional Medication

A large study (covering 2,400 CBD oil users) by Brightfield Group showed that approximately half of the people who used CBD stopped taking traditional medications. According to the researchers, this study is the largest study on CBD usage and its effect on the human body. According to the study report, 80% participants said they found the CBD oil extremely effective. Participants used CBD for a variety of usages including nausea, headaches, migraines, muscle tension or strain, joint pain, inflammation, depression, anxiety, and insomnia. This (https://s3-us-west-2.amazonaws.com/hellomd-news/Understanding-Cannabidiol-CBD-Report.pdf) link will give you the summary of the study report.

Problems with traditional medicine

Traditional medications help, but they also have side effects including:

- o Allergies: Some people have strong reactions to some traditional medicines. Occasionally, these allergies can be deadly.

o   Medicine interactions: These days' people are taking two or more medications daily and this is causing a bad reaction in the patient's body. The symptoms can become serious and cause new illness.

o   Medicine-food interactions: Traditional medications can react with food. Medicine-food interactions can cause serious symptoms.

o   Overmedication: If you are not careful, you might overdose on medication and trigger a fatal reaction. This situation is especially dangerous for kids and older adults.

o   Addiction: Long-term use of traditional medication can cause dependency. This is a serious problem in today's America.

In contrast, you avoid all these side effects by using CBD oil.

CBD truly works. Let's discuss how to cure diseases and relieve pain with CBD Hemp Oil:

Scientifically proven benefits of the CBD

1. CBD Fights Against Cancer: Studies show (http://www.tandfonline.com/doi/abs/10.1080/13543784.2016.1236913; https://www.ncbi.nlm.nih.gov/pmc/articles/PMC5009497/; https://www.ncbi.nlm.nih.gov/pmc/articles/PMC5009497/) that CBD has an antitumor effect and could be used to improve standard cancer treatments. There are instances where CBD successfully halted the growth of cancer cells. CBD can also increase the rate of tumor cell death in colon and leukemia cancer patients. CBD is an antitumor agent and it can decrease human glioma cell growth and invasion. Anticancer mechanisms of CBD:

   - CBD decreases cancer cell proliferation by blocking CPR55 signaling.

   - CBD activates lymphokine (LAK) and helps kill cancer cells better.

   - CBD cause the cancer cells to die by decreasing their ability.

2. Relieves Pain and Inflammation: According to studies (https://www.ncbi.nlm.nih.gov/pubmed/17257464/; https://www.ncbi.nlm.nih.gov/pubmed/22585736), CBD is useful in pain modulation by inhibiting neural

transmission in pain pathways. CBD is anti-inflammatory and acts as a therapeutic agent for a variety of pain and inflammatory associated disorders. CBD suppresses neuropathic pain and chronic inflammation in patients. CBD binds to the CB1 receptors to relieve pain throughout your body. CBD is even a promising tool treating prostate and breast cancer.

3. CBD Relieves Nausea and increases appetite: Study shows (https://www.ncbi.nlm.nih.gov/pubmed/21827451) CBD relieve nausea and vomiting. Data (https://www.cancer.gov/about-cancer/treatment/cam/hp/cannabis-pdq#section/all) provided by the National Cancer Institute shows that CBD increased appetite.

4. CBD Reduces Anxiety: Studies show (https://www.ncbi.nlm.nih.gov/pubmed/22729452; https://www.ncbi.nlm.nih.gov/pubmed/20829306/; https://www.ncbi.nlm.nih.gov/pubmed/22290374) CBD reduces various types of anxiety, including social anxiety, obsessive-compulsive disorder, panic disorder, and other types of stress disorder.

5. CBD May Relieve Multiple Sclerosis Symptoms: Studies show (https://www.ncbi.nlm.nih.gov/pubmed

/18035205;
https://www.ncbi.nlm.nih.gov/pubmed/17355549;
https://www.ncbi.nlm.nih.gov/pubmedhealth/PMH0025286/) that CBD may relieve symptoms in multiple sclerosis patients.

6. CBD Helps with Epileptic Seizures: Studies show (https://www.ncbi.nlm.nih.gov/pubmed/7413719; https://www.ncbi.nlm.nih.gov/pmc/articles/PMC4157067/; https://www.ncbi.nlm.nih.gov/pmc/articles/PMC4157067/) that CBD is a promising therapy for epilepsy treatment. Studies show after CBD treatment, children experienced better mood, increased alertness, and improved sleep. Studies also show 39% children had a 50% reduction in seizures.

7. CBD is Beneficial in Rheumatoid Arthritis: Study shows (https://www.ncbi.nlm.nih.gov/pubmed/16023222?dopt=Abstract) CBD is anti-inflammatory and provide relief of joint pain and swelling and decrease joint. CBD also decrease joint destruction and disease progression.

8. Controls Diabetes: Study shows (https://www.organicfacts.net/ways-diabetes-control.html?utm_source=internal&utm_medium=link&utm_campaign=smar

tlinks) that CBD oil can lower the level of insulin and control diabetes.

9. Skin Care: Study shows (https://www.ncbi.nlm.nih.gov/pmc/articles/PMC4151231/) the usage of CBD oil can reduce the signs and symptoms of acne and eczema. The oil can also soothe itchiness, redness and swollen areas of the skin.

10. Boost Immune System: Study shows (http://www.sciencedirect.com/science/article/pii/S0028390807001888) that CBD oil can help regulate overactive immune systems.

11. Promotes Heart Health: Study shows (https://www.ncbi.nlm.nih.gov/pubmed/22670794) that CBD oil is also beneficial for the cardiovascular system. The oil heals the damage done by inflammation.

Chapter 3 Potential Side Effects of CBD

Using CBD has many benefits, but the oil is not all good and well in every single case. Some people can feel a few side effects and they vary from one person to another. The most common adverse effects of CBD oil:

- A Dry Mouth: A dry mouth is one of the most common side effects of using CBD oil. This particular side effect is caused by activity that the oil has on the nervous system of the user. The symptom is also known as the cotton mouth. It will only make you thirsty.

- Reduced Blood Pressure: Reduction in blood pressure levels is another side effect of using CBD oil. However, for hypertension patients, this reduction is not considered a side effect, since the oil will act as a treatment for high blood pressure. An important fact to remember, CBD will only cause your blood pressure to go down if you take it in high doses and high concentrations. So, basically, you are safe from this side effect.

- Lightheadedness: A drop in blood pressure can cause Lightheadedness. This side effect is temporary and you can resolve it by drinking a cup of tea or coffee.

- Drowsiness: Unlike the THC, CBD doesn't cause any feeling of 'high'. In most cases, CBD is a wake-inducing agent, but it can cause drowsiness in some users. Drowsiness is nothing serious and should go away on its own.

- o Can cause a problem for Parkinson's disease patients: High doses of CBD oil use in Parkinson's disease patients can worsen tremor and muscle movement. So consult with your doctor before taking CBD.

- o Inhibition of hepatic drug metabolism: CBD can interact with a few traditional medications. So, consult with your doctor before using CBD if you are taking traditional medication.

Contraindications

Consult with your physician if you have been diagnosed with or are at high risk of developing any of the following disorders:

- o Immune or autoimmune disorder

- o High blood pressure, heart disease, angina or arrhythmia

- o Severe depression, bipolar disorder or schizophrenia

The U.S. Food and Drug Administration (FDA) has yet to approve the CBD for any condition.

Chapter 4 Is CBD Oil Legal?

There are two types of Cannabidiol available for you to purchase. One is extracted from industrially grown hemp plants and another is medical marijuana plants. Both are different Cannabis, but grown for different purposes, so their legal status is also different. To get medical marijuana, you need to live in certain states and obtain a prescription from a doctor.

CBD from Medical Marijuana

Medical marijuana plants are grown to be high in CBD and they also contain varying amounts of THC. THC, as you know makes you 'high". This type of CBD is prescribed by doctors and sold at licensed dispensaries for particular health conditions in countries where marijuana is regulated – like the US. This type of CBD is not currently legal everywhere in the United States because of the existence of THC.

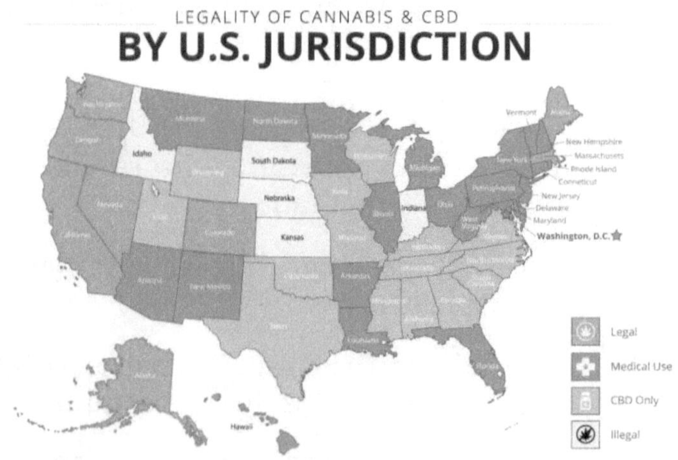

CBD from Industrial Hemp

The FDA of the United States considers hemp oil CBD as a dietary supplement because they are made from industrial hemp plants. So good news for you is, if you live in the U.S. you can legally purchase and consume CBD made from industrial hemp plants. The industrial hemp plant extracted CBD doesn't make you 'high'. The federal governments ruling is "every CBD products containing less than 0.3% THC is legal in the U.S.

CBD legality around the world

CBD is legal in most countries as a prescription drug. However, purchasing it as a dietary supplement is a different story. The following table shows the current status of non-prescription CBD legality in various countries. If your country is not included in the table, then most probably you will need a prescription for CBD. Most European countries allow CBD oils that contain less than 0.2% THC.

Non-prescription CBD Legality by Country

Country	Status
UK	legal
Australia	illegal
Brazil	illegal
Canada	illegal
China	illegal
France	illegal
Germany	illegal
Japan	legal
Netherlands	legal
New Zealand	illegal
Russia	illegal
Slovakia	illegal
Switzerland	legal

<u>Chapter 5 CBD Buying Guide</u>

In this chapter, we are going to discuss what to consider when buying CBD. Whether you want to buy CBD capsules, tinctures, oil or topical, it is important to know what you are looking for. The following are some clarification and guidance so you can buy top quality CBD.

CBD volume vs Hemp volume

The first thing you should look for is how much CBD is in a product. Make sure the product label clearly states its quantity of hemp oil and CBD volume levels.

Concentration of CBD

Each CBD product should clearly mention its certain concentration amount. The CBD concentration determines the strength of the product.

Ingredients and processing you should look for

- Always check the purity, it should be 50% CBD or more

- Pesticide/Herbicide free

- 100% organic

- No chemical fertilizers

- Non-GMO

- PCR Distillate or Full Spectrum Oil

- o   Third party lab test results

- o   CO2 extraction method

- o   Ingredient percentages

- o   Flavoring/ natural terpenes

- o   Cutting agent MCT (Coconut Oil)

- o   Winterized (optional)

- o   Buy CBD products manufactured in the U.S. or Canada. Strict regulations guarantee high quality.

- o   Remember, high-quality CBD oil should cost at least $40 to $50.

CBD Dosing

As a beginner, you should start with a standard adult dose of 1 to 2 mg daily. CBD works best when used regularly, so take CBD just like a daily supplement or vitamin. After one week of use, you should know the appropriate dosage for you. Here are some recommendations:

- o   Treatment for Epilepsy: 200 to 300 mg CBD by mouth daily

- o   Treatment for Schizophrenia: 40 to 1,280 mg CBD by mouth daily

- o   Treatment for Glaucoma: 20 to 40 mg applied under the tongue daily

- o Treatment for sleep disorders: 40 to 160 mg CBD by mouth daily

- o Treatment for chronic pain: 2.5 to 20 mg CBD by mouth daily

- o Treatment for movement problems: 10 mg by mouth daily

- o General health and wellness: 2.5 to 15 mg CBD by mouth daily

Different types of CBD products

You can use CBD a variety of ways, including

CBD Vaporizer

CBD is popular for those who want to "smoke" their CBD oil. CBD vaporizers work similar to an e-cigarette. You heat up one end and inhale through the other end. The features:

- o Reusable battery

- o Highest CBD absorption

- o Quickest reaction

- o Safe for the lungs and easy to use

- o Good for systemic internal ailments

CBD Topical

CBD topical absorbs through the skin and mixes into the bloodstream quickly. People with lifelong medical conditions such as fibromyalgia, epilepsy, MS, and cancer can benefit from CBD topical –balms, lotions, creams, and lotions. The features:

- o   Promotes healthy skin

- o   Eases stiffness

- o   Reduce inflammation of arthritis

- o   Good for localized pain in muscles/joints

CBD Gummies and Edibles

Gummies are a fun way to get your CBD. It is popular for consumers who don't like swallowing pills and capsules. The features:

- o   Difficult to dose

- o   Takes longer to work

- o   Lasts the longest

- o   Good for systemic internal ailments

- o   Low bioavailability (4% to 12%)

CBD Tinctures

Tinctures are the easiest and effective ways to get your CBD. You can even add them to a drink, recipe or baked goods. However, many prefer the pure form. The features:

- Good for people who can't vape
- Easy to digest
- Long lasting

CBD Capsules

Capsules are an easy way to consume your CBD. They are odorless, tasteless and excellent options for travel.

CBD Oil Concentrates

CBD oil concentrate is usually the strongest type of CBD. CBD oil concentrates are taken sublingually as a tincture. You can put it in a vaporizer or add to your food.

Things to avoid

- Claims of curing diseases without evidence
- Hidden subscriptions

- o   Pyramid scheme companies

- o   Plastic cartridges full of BPA

- o   Extracted with alcohol/ethanol

- o   Artificial flavoring

- o   Hemp oil with no CBD

- o   Harmful cutting agents such as PEG, Vegetable Glycerin, Propylene Glycol

Tips for buying CBD Oil online

With so many choices, buying CBD oil online can be a difficult and confusing process. Here are a few tips to make things easier for you:

- o   Avoid free trial bottle of CBD: Some online sellers will offer you a free trial bottle of CBD. You only have to pay a small shipping and handling fee. The catch is they will send you a very low-quality product. Importantly, these companies will continue to charge your credit card every month until you cancel your "subscription". This is a scam and beware of this type of trial offer.

- o   Make sure you are buying the right product: Buy only CBD oil and don't get fooled by hemp seed oil.

- o   Buy from a reputable brand: Buy your CBD oil from a reputable brand. A third party lab report is essential to ensure quality.

o   Read reviews: Read product reviews on the product page and on the company's Facebook page. Also, you can join a "CBD oil users group".

Chapter 6 How to Cure Diseases and Relieve Pain with CBD Oil

In this chapter, we are going to discuss how the CBD Oil can help you with a variety of diseases. Before starting, we are going to talk about CBD dosage calculator.

The following three sites will help you calculate your CBD dosage:

1. https://honestmarijuana.com/cbd-dosage-calculator/

2. https://vitaleafnaturals.com/pages/cbd-oil-drops-dosage-calculator

3. https://www.cbdoilusers.com/cbd-oil-drops-dosage-calculator/

Standard dosing recommendations for CBD oil

o Start your first day by taking 1 drop of CBD oil

o Increase amount to 2 drops daily during the first 3 to 4 weeks or until you feel better.

o Don't take your drops all at once. Spread them evenly throughout your day.

o If you do not feel better after 3 to 4 weeks of usage, increase the dosage.

o   Experiment a little to know what works for you.

Let's start with disease cure:

CBD for Anxiety

Anxiety is a serious mental health concern in the U.S. Data shows that about 66 million U.S. adults have an anxiety disorder. CBD is an effective anxiety treatment, (https://www.ncbi.nlm.nih.gov/pubmed/2634 1731), but only a few uses CBD as an anxiety treatment.

CBD oil dosage for anxiety

If you are taking CBD tincture, then take 5 mg tincture 1 to 3 times daily. Start with 1 to 3 drops. Place it under your tongue for 1 minute and then swallow.

If you prefer pills, then take 1 to 3 CBD capsules daily. You need a few days to find out the ideal CBD dosage for your body.

Start with the above mention dosage and if you don't experience enough relief within a few days, then go for a higher dosage. For example, 30 to 37.5 mg CBD for the first 3 to 4 days to manage severe anxiety. Once you feel calmer, you can go back to the low CBD dosage. Pure CBD is not toxic and wouldn't cause fatality even if taken in a large dosage

(https://www.ncbi.nlm.nih.gov/pubmed/2212
9319).

CBD oil for Back Pain

CBD inhibits neuronal transmission in the pain
pathways of your body. It reduces inflammation
and stops back pain. Whether you apply CBD on
the skin, ingest or drink it, the result is
essentially same. The difference is how targeted
you wanted the pain relief to be.

Dosage

The most common way of applying the oil is to
place a few drops under your tongue and
swallow it. The fastest onset of effects will be
from sublingual tinctures and inhalation.
Rubbing a few drops of CBD directly onto your
sore spots is another simple way. You may need
assistance from others, but it is an effective
option. If topical or sublingual is not your thing,
then you can cook with CBD oil instead. Many
patients like to combine different methods to
get more benefits. Start out with low doses and
increase the dose in even increments slowly
until you reach your desired effect. After a
couple of days, you can increase your dosage. A
low starting dosage is 5 to 10 mg CBD.

CBD oil for Chronic Pain

Data shows that 10% of the world population is suffering from chronic pain on a daily basis.

CBD oil dosage for chronic pain

As mentioned before, start with a small dosage. If you are using vaporizing, then start with 1 to 10 seconds of inhaling and wait 3 minutes for the oil to work. If you are taking it by mouth, then take 5 to 20 mg CBD for about 25 days.

CBD for Depression

More than 16 million people in the U.S. suffer from depression. Currently about 13% of the U.S., the population is taking some type of antidepressant. CBD is a powerful cure to treat any type of depression.

CBD oil dosage for Depression

The daily dosage of CBD is important to alleviate depression. As a beginner, you should use 25 to 50 mg daily and increase gradually. Depression affects the patients' eating habits, so you can mix CBD product with your food.

Acne

An acne is a form of skin disease affecting the oil glands in the skin. CBD can treat serious skin conditions, including eczema, psoriasis and it can make you look younger.

Dosage

Clean your skin and massage 2 pumps of CBD enriched face cream into your face and neck. You can take 1 to 2 drops of CBD oil before going to bed.

Asthma

During an asthma attack, the air passageways in the mouth and nose become constricted. This causes the oxygen flow to restricted severely. Using CBD oil can help to open up these airways. More than 75% asthma patients also experience chest pain and CBD also provide pain relief.

Dosage

Doctors recommend that patients should understand how their bodies work and take CBD accordingly. For a quick relief, you can use a vaporizer or tincture. Both of them are much gentler on your body and deliver without irritation. However, if vaporizer makes you cough, then an edible or tincture is best for you. As an edible, take 3 drops under your tongue 3 times daily.

Bipolar Disorder

CBD oil is a natural bipolar disorder treatment. Taking CBD can help you slowly reduce your bipolar pharmaceutical medication.

Dosage

You can vaporize or take it orally. You can take 0.5 ml CBD in the morning and 1 ml at night before sleep.

Diabetes

Data (http://www.letfreedomgrow.com/cmu/diabetes_5.htm) shows that CBD can prevent diabetic complications like cell inflammation, cell damage and build up of plaque in arteries. CBD can stabilize a person's blood sugars and reduce inflammation that is found in many diabetics.

Dosage

CBD dosages can range from 10 mg to 200 mg per day. Start slowly with 10 mg two times daily and increase dosages later.

Fibromyalgia

Fibromyalgia is a chronic disorder that causes fatigue, cognitive issues, and pain.

Dosage

You can use vaping or smoking. The effects last for about 3 hours. Edibles take longer to work but can give you 6 hours of pain relief. Topical and oil extracts are other options for you.

Glaucoma

Glaucoma is an eye condition that causes damage to the optic nerve. CBD has been well known to treat eye pressure associated with glaucoma. Studies done on treating glaucoma with CBD shows the promising result.

Dosage

Start with lowest recommended dosage, 2 drops. Then increase, as you feel comfortable. Dosing twice-daily morning and evening is normally sufficient.

Irritable Bowel Syndrome

Irritable Bowel Syndrome can cause stomach cramps, bloating, constipation and/or diarrhea. Scientists have proven that CBD can successfully heal IBS.

Dosage

You can take CBD vaporizers, capsules or edibles. Start with a low dosage of 200 mg and go for a higher dosage.

Cancer

Cancer patients can use CBD and CBD ointments as chemo alternative. Cannabinoids are not only antioxidant phytonutrients but powerful "herbal chemo" agents. CBD is a potent medicine against tumor growth.

Dosage

It is recommended, that an average person should ingest about 60 grams or 60 ml CBD oil treatment. Start with three doses per day. Early in the morning, in the afternoon and an hour before bed.

Chapter 7 CBD Oil Recipes for Beginners

Before we start the recipes, let's know how you can make canna-oil at home very easily!

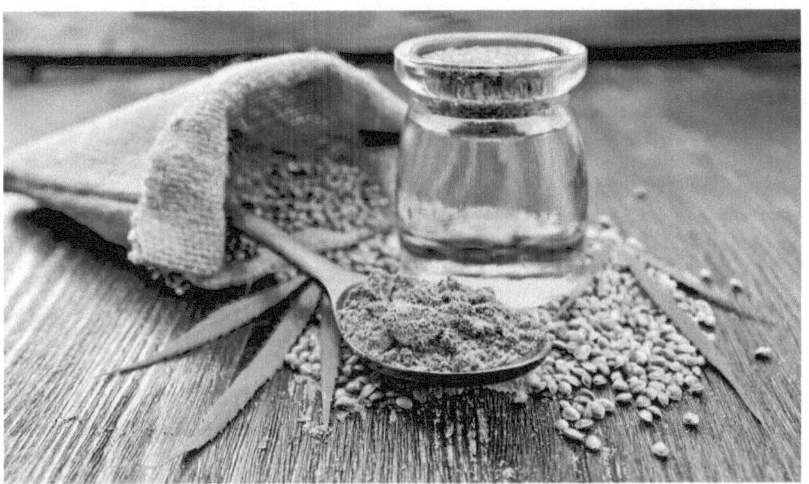

Cannabis or Canna-oil

Ingredients

- o   Potent marijuana – 1 ounce
- o   Oil – 2 cups

Method

1. Grind the cannabis. Do not grind the cannabis to a fine powder.

2. In a slow cooker, combine oil and cannabis. Heat on low heat or warm for few hours. Stir occasionally.

3. Add a small amount of water to avoid burning.

4. Strain and store the oil. Do not squeeze the cheesecloth.

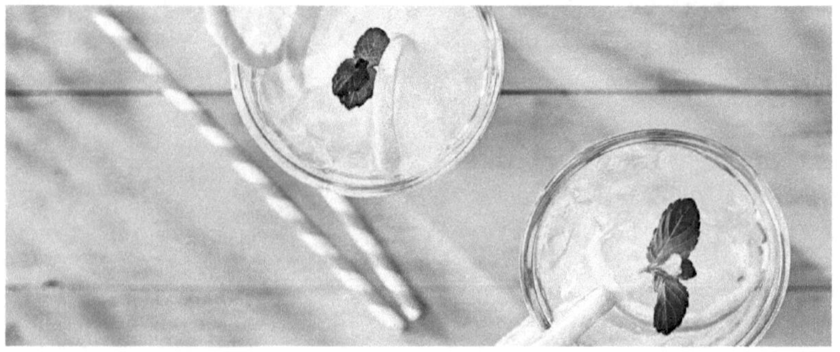

CBD-Infused Lemonade

Ingredients for 6 servings

- o   Juice of 6 to 8 lemons

- o   Sugar – 1 cup

- o   Water – 5 cups

- o   Seltzer – 1 cup

- o   Fresh mint – 1 bunch

- o   CBD oil- 6 tsp.

Method

1. Heat 1 cup water and 1 cup sugar in a pan over medium heat. Stir and dissolve the sugar. Set aside the pan and cool completely.

2. Add the lemon juice to the serving glasses and place a few basil leaves.

3. Add remaining water, CBD, sugar mixture to the lemon juice. Stir to mix.

4. Fill the glasses ¾ with lemonade, then fill the rest with seltzer water.

5. Serve.

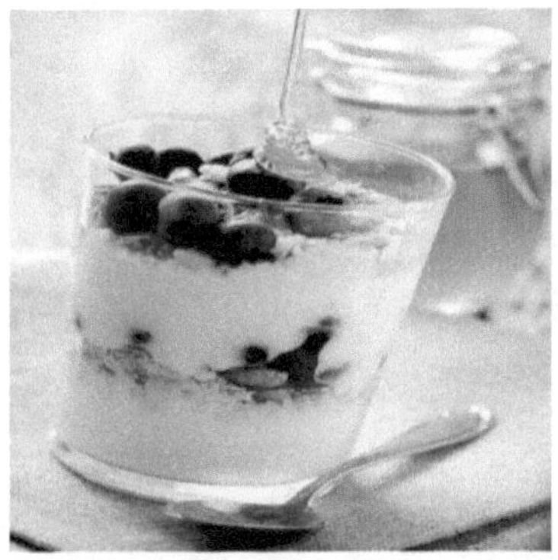

CBD Yogurt Blueberry Parfait

Ingredients 1 serving

- o   Fresh blueberries – 6 ounces

- o   Greek yogurt – 2/3 cup

- o   Granola – ½ cup

- o   Honey – 2 tbsp.

- o   Pinch of salt and cinnamon
- o   CBD oil – ¾ tsp.

Method

1. Place CBD and honey in a double-boiler at low heat and blend. Set aside.

2. In another bowl, mix yogurt with cinnamon and salt.

3. Add the yogurt mix at the bottom of the glass, then layer half of the granola.

4. Top with half blueberries. Then drizzle with CBD infused honey.

5. Repeat the four layers and serve.

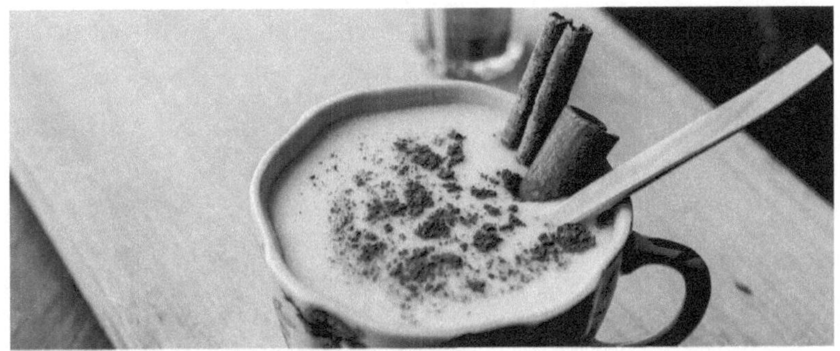

CBD-Infused Eggnog

Ingredients for 16 servings

- o Eggs – 8, separated

- o Sugar – 1/3 cup

- o Salt – ½ tsp.

- o Whole milk – 4 cups

- o Heavy whipping cream – 2 cups

- o Freshly grated cinnamon or nutmeg – 1 tsp. plus more for garnish

- o Vanilla extract – 1 tsp.

- o CBD oil – ¾ tsp. per mug

Method

1. Whisk together the sugar, salt and egg yolks until smooth.

2. Add the vanilla, nutmeg, whipping cream and whole milk. Whisk again until smooth.

3. Whisk the egg whites for 4 minutes or until soft peaks form.

4. Fold the whipped egg whites into the cream mixture until smooth.

5. Chill until cold.

6. Add ¾ tsp. CBD to each serving. Top with nutmeg and garnish with cinnamon sticks.

7. Serve.

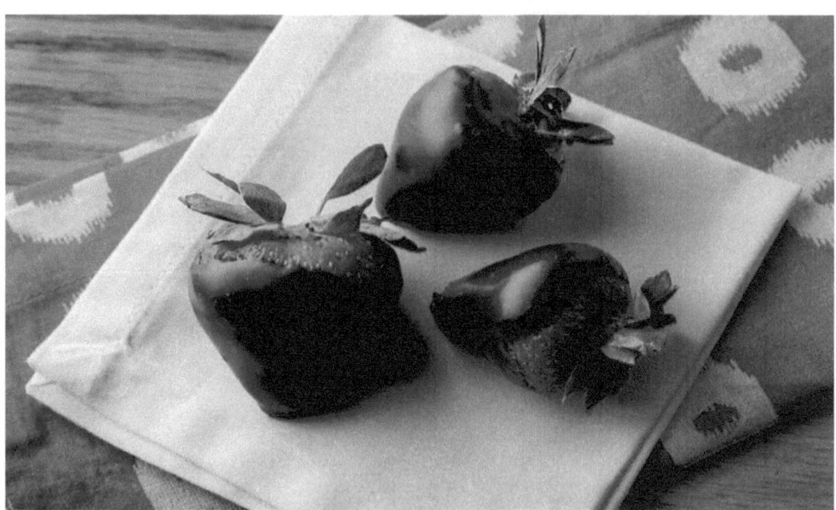

Dessert Strawberries

Ingredients for 4 servings

- o CBD oil – 2 tbsp.

- o Chocolate chips – 1 ½ cups

- o Strawberries with stems – 12

Method

1. Stir together CBD oil and chocolate chips in a microwave-safe bowl. Heat in the microwave in 15-second intervals until smooth and melted. Stir until chocolate reaches room temperature.

2. Dip the berries into the melted chocolate.

3. Place on the parchment paper and leave alone for 30 minutes.

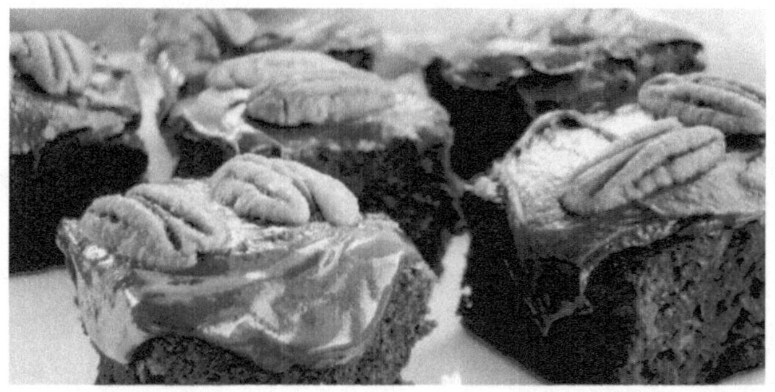

Delicious Pecan Brownies

Ingredients for 24 servings

- o   Cooking spray
- o   Your favorite boxed brownie mix
- o   CBD oil − 1/3 cup

- o   Water – 1/3 cup

- o   Eggs – 2 large, lightly brown

- o   Semisweet chocolate chips – ½ cup

- o   Roasted and glazed pecans – ¼ cup, crushed

- o   Melted chocolate

- o   Crushed health bar

Method

1. Preheat the oven to 340F. Lightly grease a 9 x 13-inch brownie pan with cooking spray.

2. In a bowl, combine water, CBD oil, and eggs.

3. Slowly stir the brownie mix until blended.

4. Add the pecans and chocolate chips. Into the prepared baking pan, spread the batter evenly.

5. Bake until a toothpick inserted into the center of the brownies comes out clean. Follow the package directions.

6. Remove and let cool for 30 minutes.

7. Cut into 24 equal pieces.

8. Melt the chocolate in the microwave.

9. Dip the brownie in the chocolate and coat them evenly with chocolate. Place on parchment paper and repeat the process with the remaining brownies.

10. Sprinkle the health bar crumbles on top of the brownies and serve.

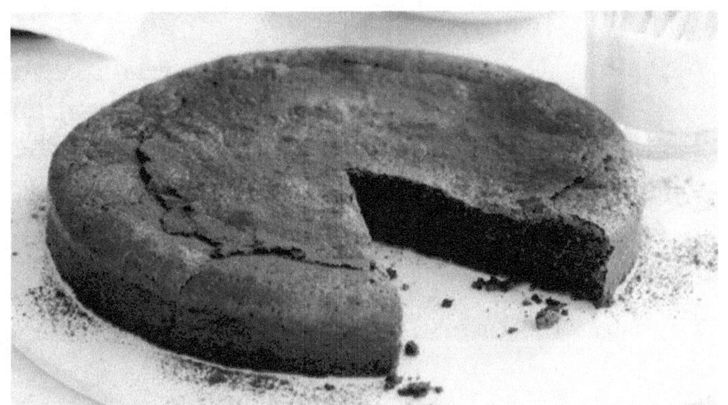

Flourless Chocolate Cake

Ingredients for 8 slices

- o   Semisweet chocolate – 12 ounces

- o   CBD-infused butter – 12 tbsp.

- o   Fine salt – ¼ tsp.

- o   Large eggs – 6, room temperature

- o   Granulated sugar – 1.5 cups

- o   Cocoa powder and confectioners' sugar for dusting – 1 tbsp.

Method

1. Preheat the oven to 325F. Grease a 9 x 2-inch springform pan with cooking spray.

2. In a heatproof bowl, put the butter and chocolate. Melt in the microwave.

3. Beat the sugar and eggs with a whisk for 8 to 10 minutes or until light and thickened. Fold the melted chocolate into the whipped eggs until mixed evenly.

4. Pour the batter into the prepared pan and bake for 1 hour and 25 minutes, or until a toothpick inserted into the middle of the cake comes out wet, but not gooey. Remove and cool on a wire rack.

5. Dust cooled cake with cocoa powder and confectioners' sugar. Serve.

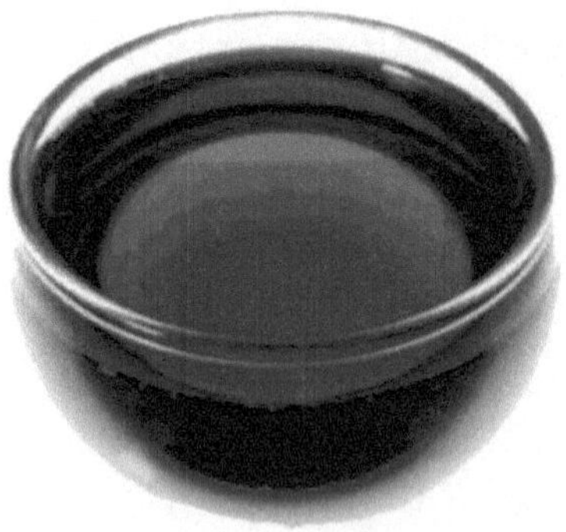

Super Potent Homemade CBD Oil Recipe

Ingredients

- o Ground and dried trim or shake 100g or ground buds 30g (from the most potent CBD strains)

- o Grain alcohol – 4L or 190 proof alcohol

Equipment

- o Double boiler

- o Plastic syringe

- o Funnel

- o Wooden spoon

- o Silicon spatula

- o Catchment container

- o Mason jar

- o Cheesecloth or sieve

- o Electric Stove

- o Glass or ceramic mixing bowl

Method

1. Make sure your work area and all your equipment are clean.

2 . Soak the cannabis in the alcohol. Use a wooden spoon to stir and remove the resin. Leave overnight.

3 . Filter the mixture into the catchment container in the morning. Leaving out as much liquid as you can.

4 . Pour the extracted liquid into a double boiler.

5 . Heat over very low heat until bubbles form. Evaporate all the alcohol on low heat. It could take about 20 to 30 minutes.

6 . Don't allow the mixture to get too hot. Keep stirring to mix in some air.

7 . Use the spatula to mix the solution and scrape the bowl.

8 . Now carefully transfer the concentrated oil into a storage bottle or a dosage container before it cools off and becomes too thick.

Remember, the potency of your CBD oil depends on the raw material you use.

Conclusion

Have you tried all the pills, potions and drugs but are still dealing with pains, aches, physical discomforts, and diseases? Do you want to learn how to cure your body naturally? Then forgot the prescription drugs and start using CBD. Studies on CBD's natural health benefits are extensive and new beneficial aspects of the CBD are revealing every day. This book gives you the information you need to know about CBD oil and how to make it work for you. Written in easy to understand language, this book contains the answers you have been looking for. The book even shows you how to make your own CBD oil and make things easier for you. Start using the CBD oil today and feel the difference within days!

9 781724 431738